IMAGINATIONPRESS

AND I DON'T
SURRENDER
to STIGMAS and JUDGMENTS

MIRIAM WHITEHEAD-BRICE

Editors

Teresa Hamilton

Phillip Wizeman

Cover & Layout Artist

Francis Adams

Publisher

Imagination Press, LLC

And I Don't Surrender (AIDS)
to Stigmas and Judgements
by Miriam Whitehead-Brice

First Edition

Printed in the United States of America

ISBN 978-0-9995209-6-3

Copyright© 2018

CONTENTS

Dedication

This is dedicated to those whose
voice will never be heard and their story never
told. This is also dedicated to those who think that
their pain will never end.
There is

LIFE AFTER DIAGNOSIS

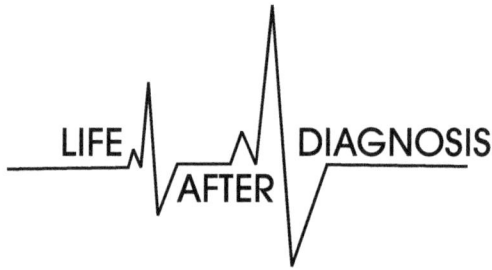

Do not let HIV/AIDS discourage you.
This story is not just about HIV/AIDS! This story will reveal parts of
life that a lot of people keep in the closet. You can not heal what you
do not say. Whispers only
widen the secrets. Turned heads exhaust and heighten
the myths; and closed minds ignore the threats and
complications of diseases.

Prologue

This is a book of my memoirs. I wrote this book for freedom's sake. It is also for that person who thinks that there is no hope in their situation.

I am encouraging someone for life. Be a productive member of society, and please know, whatever you go through in life should not affect your purpose. It should refine it. I am an example of "Life After Diagnosis." I have been through some rough times but, the word "through" means there's an exit.

Living with multiple diagnoses can be overwhelming.

- Getting prescriptions and dealing with the side effects. Keeping up with medication adherence and doctor appointments
- Staying mentally stable in order to function properly. I have many hats and keep the baggage low; a Wife, Mother, Grandmother, Minister, Chaplain, HIV/AIDS Activist, Poet, and Support groups member.

Be confident; live on purpose. You can because, I do!

AIDS
And I Don't Surrender
to Stigmas and Judgments

Visit my website:
www. miriamwbrice.com

"And they overcame him by the blood of the Lamb and by the word of their testimony, and they did not love their lives to the death" (Revelation 12.11).

INTRODUCTION

Roots Exposed

I drove past a tree and saw that its roots were exposed. The roots were mangled and tangled, but you could clearly see the tree's growth. I wondered, what if people saw others with their roots exposed? Would they embrace each other, or see the person approaching, and then walk past them? Maybe if our roots were visible, our testimonies could not hide. People would be able to see, understand, and recover because, hope is right before their eyes. Loneliness would not be so prevalent, and judging would not be so easy. People would see that their transgressions and another's offenses would be relatable evils. If our past was shown first, most of us would attempt to mask those regretful times. Then we would realize that the past matured us. It created a definite need to better our lives. Being exposed should welcome victory.

CHAPTER
ONE

Roots Exposed Continued

I ignored boundaries. I recall my mother telling me that when I learned to crawl, I would constantly crawl off something and hit the floor. My father said I had horrible table manners as a toddler. They placed mats and newspaper under my highchair before giving me food in a separate room. I ate what I wanted and then the rest of the food would go in my hair, on the chair, on the floor, and on my clothes. It was definitely bath time after meals!   My aunt told me that I was mean to my brother and sister. By the time I was enrolled in school, my family moved from Baltimore, Maryland to Harrisburg, Pennsylvania because my Father was an executive who traveled for his job. He inspected the products that his company made. He traveled the world. Sometimes, he would drive if it was here in the United States. At times, he brought me and my siblings gifts from wherever he went. However, we still attended church in Baltimore. I recall riding up and down I-83 at least two days a week to attend church. I also recall one cold and icy day, we were on our way to church and my father lost control of the car. He hit a patch of ice and we headed towards an embankment; I remember something lifting the car and placing it safely upon a small hill. This was my first recollection of Angels!   My memories of that particular stretch of highway were not very pleasant because, of the constant back and forth. I could smell the bakery and the vinegar plant on the way to Baltimore.

We lived in Harrisburg during my years from kindergarten to third grade. I was the only black girl in my class. I realized in first grade that I was different from my classmates during a Halloween party. I did not understand why the teacher recognized me in a costume. I went home, stared into the mirror, and went over the whole memory of that Halloween party. I noticed my wrist, hands, face, and neck were darker than the white Barbie doll mask and costume. I never questioned it; I was just aware of my differences. Back in Baltimore during fourth grade, the class was asked to write a poem. Feeling as if I was at the bottom of the totem pole, because of my unexplainable mood swings. I wrote my first poem, "I Wish I Was a Butterfly." I received an "A" on this project. This was the start of me expressing myself through poetry. I felt better writing things out.

I Wish I Was a Butterfly

I wish I were a butterfly flying through the air;
then everyone below would look up to me and stare.
I wish I were a butterfly high above the ground;
then all of the ants would look up to me and frown.
Look at me, look at me, I'm flying through the air.
I have no concerns and I'm pretty and without a care.
I am a butterfly and I'm the only one
who looks at herself and likes herself.
I'm getting things done.

Miriam Whitehead - 9 years old

I was very curious about some things. One day I saw my mom writing a check. The way my parents wrote checks and snatched them out of the checkbook on the perforated lines seemed fun. I took one of my mother's check books to school. I wrote all of my classmates one-thousand-dollar checks. Then I wrote my teacher a check for a million dollars. The teacher called my mother. When I got home, I had to hold my hands out while she beat them with a wooden brush; palms up.

I was not the kindest sister to my two siblings, a brother and sister, but having fun was always my goal. I was often manipulative and creative as a child. Some Christmases and birthdays I would wrap up dirty underwear, or personals of theirs I had burned and/or broken as gifts for them. I convinced my sister to get in the dryer without closing the door. I was able to just push the little button inside the door to make it go around. I also convinced her to stand in the washing machine during the spin cycle. I convinced my brother to be the ramp we needed for our bikes to jump over. He ended up in the hospital when I dared him to ride his bike down the stairs. I was never bored. My mom and dad were getting weary from my odd ways. They gave me alternatives, so I backed off. I received two out of the three strikes allotted me. It may have been three or more, I just spread them out. I realized when I got older that they just gave me chances because of the Lord!

My play time included playing with bugs and finding new ways to mutilate and kill them. Hurting other animals such as mice, turtles, rabbits, and birds peaked my curiosity. I would tug and cut on them until their death. When a mouse was caught on a sticky trap I would kill it, slowly. When I caught water bugs, cockroaches, grasshoppers, and lightening bugs, I would try different ways to torture them. Putting spiders and water bugs in a jar and watching them fight was the highlight of my day. My sister and brother did not want to play those games; so, playing by myself was easy. I did not need to be by myself, but, I liked being by myself! My mother said that I had a problem and it was not a good idea for me to have pets. My warped sense of humor seemed attractive to those whose humor was also a bit slanted and on the edge of scary! As a pre-teen, I decided that my father should divorce my mother because of how she would beat me and my siblings. I would cause arguments between them. Then I would side with my father and intervene. I would pick a subject and get them fussing about it.

My mom was aware of my actions. I did not care, that just fueled the fire and I would get happier. My sister and brother would get mad at me. Physical punishments introduced me to manipulating hatred. The punishments and corrections for my actions seemed too harsh. Self-mutilation became interesting. I would peel the hangnails from one my fingers down to the first knuckle or digit, I would stick huge safety pins in the calluses in the bottom of my feet, I placed my tongue on the insides of the freezer and would snatch it off quickly (my tongue would bleed). When I would get those little white bumps on my tongue, lie bumps, I would strategically cut them off with a toe nail clipper. Sometimes I missed, and my tongue would bleed but, that just made me more determined to find that bump! Picking scabs gave me pleasure, but, only the slightly healed scabs. Somehow the pain felt good.

I promised myself that when I had children, punishments and correction would not be as degrading and unreasonable as I had experienced as a child. Raising a child in fear is different because, the outcome could cause disrespectfulness, hatred, and other mental issues and insecurities. I repeated a lot of things that I got beatings for, so at one point I was not afraid of the consequences until that moment of "take off your clothes," or "hold your hands out." The most hateful feelings came when my mom would ask me to come to her so that she could put a band-aid or some medicinal ointment on the lashes, bruises, or cuts. I would pretend to be sorrowful. Why was she this way? Who had hurt my mommy so harshly as to make her hurt me? Was this happening to other kids? No one tells?

Grandparents

Could my mother's actions be generational? Was she just mean? Did she know any better? These are things I wondered about. I envied kids who just got punished verbally. My mom's mother passed away when my mom was young. Her father was an abusive, cussing, smoking, drunkard. I heard the horror stories of what my mother and her brothers endured. Evidently, she forgave him. She would pick him up and bring him to our house. He seemed to carry evil on him like a shroud. I did not understand why she wanted him around. Maybe it was therapy for her; but it was not therapy for me! As a matter of fact, it was clarity! The stench of cigarettes on him was so strong; it seemed as if he carried ashes in his pockets instead of lint. I touched his face and the tiny, but seen, gray hairs almost pricked my fingers. He was frail, and his clothes were a size too big. I was disgusted by the very thought of him abusing my mother. I recalled the previous beatings she gave me and pictured his face in the place of my mother's. I could not control my hatred of him. I would ask my mother why she had that man in our home; she would cut her eyes at me. Maybe she forgave him. I had to repent for those thoughts of hurting him without getting caught. She did not look like him but, she probably beat me like him! She would take him and us to the Harbor. I would think of how I could push him into the water, pretend to jump in and save him, but I would drown him.

When we would visit him at his home it was smelly, dank, and narrow. He lived with a woman and her sons. I would keep swallowing my saliva, so I would not throw-up. The woman had an "I cannot wait till he dies" cloud hanging over her. I bet he never hit her! Her sons would probably kill him if he did! When he finally passed away I could not understand the sorrow and tears; I had a smirk of relief on my face. One less person that I had to pretend I liked.

When I met my paternal grandfather, he was in a wheelchair and never had a lot to say. My grandparents lived down South. I did not like going there.   At that time, outhouses and spittoons were everywhere. Their cooking made the trips a little better but watching them play chess and checkers was boring. My paternal grandmother basically had children with this man, and that was the extent of their relationship. I met her about five times. She always seemed distant and guilty, and almost never had anything to say. I wondered if she ever apologized for having sixteen children (that I know of) with different men. She was responsible for breaking up other people's families. It has been my life experience that grown adults are still living as hurtful adolescences. There were half-siblings and cousins and other relatives in close proximity without any knowledge of each other's existence. I was told by one relative that I acted like grandma when it came to having children. I thought to myself, "she would know; she did the same thing also."

Young Adulthood

My dreams were very scary. I was always dreaming of swamps, its creatures, and witches. This had an impact on my prayers and church life. Whenever I prayed I felt a witch's fingernail digging into my shoulder. So, I stopped praying for a while or would pretend to pray. I would wake up in the middle of the night and see alligators and snakes! I had dreams of falling and drowning. I had them so often that I learned how to wake from them. While I was drowning I would inhale the water and wake up.

The most vivid dream I had was of someone who was chasing me with a gun, caught me and blew my brains out; I could feel the bullet go in my head. My dreams were so real that they made me angry, moody, and tense. I needed to release my rage. I would let it out by playing board games, think of new games to play, or fuss with my siblings. Why were the dreams so bad? Who could I confide in? I knew something was wrong with the way I acted but, I watched a lot of television. I did not want to be locked up. I accepted these dreams as my fate. I was scared of the dreams and of things hissing and crawling on the floor and just accepted them as inevitable for my life.

Bedwetting became normal because, I did not want to step on the floor. It was difficult to explain this to my parents because church life was clear to them; and I did not want my thoughts of evil known to them. Eventually, the dreams became tolerable. A woman prayed for me and the witch's fingernails left. The dreams also stopped. There was such an emotional relief and release! My mother started school again. I was impressed with her endurance to meet academic goals; I would critique her papers for her. She became an evangelist at the church we frequently attended. Now I am a preacher's kid I began to like and even love my mom. One day my mom told me that it took her a long time to forgive me for the things I had done to her. My own thoughts were the same. She worked at a hospital; in my younger years. One day I said, "Mom if I showed signs, as a toddler, of ignoring boundaries, you should have imported more techniques to accommodate my ways! Then maybe I wouldn't be so curious and ignore boundaries."

During my late teens, my mom and sister were ordained as preachers. Mom also got a degree in psychology. I read some of her textbooks, I felt like my mom's patient. She started trying to diagnose me. Again, she said I was dangerous and needed help. I discovered that loving her was difficult yet, doable. She said I needed a hobby; so, she taught me how to sew with or without a pattern. That kept me more focused on things that made sense –to her! I took piano lessons also. My hair and makeup were a hobby too.   My father was a deacon, Sunday school teacher, and Trustee at the church. His job had him traveling the world from my youth and into my adulthood. He still found time to teach me how to play chess and checkers. He was also the President of the PTA in every school I attended.

My behavior at schools was just acceptable enough to keep me out of the principal's office, but not on the honor role. I started playing the clarinet in fifth grade until the eleventh grade. In high school I learned to write music and lyrics, musicality became second-nature to me. High School was not my best time mentally. I felt like a sore thumb. I was not allowed to hang out with the school kids; and the church kids made me feel uncomfortable at times and I could not hang around them a lot either. They knew I was sociable and silly.

I was baptized in Jesus' name, and received the gift of tongues, yet I questioned rules and my relationship with God; I was focused on rules and not relationship. Pretending that things were okay with both groups of people, meaning school acquaintances and the church, was easy. It was also a headache. My sense of humor and lack of vocal filters made me easy to be liked and disliked. Somehow, I was also compassionate. I was in the school band. I was in the school choir for two years, and the church choir for 20 years. Academically, I needed more attention but, still managed to graduate on time. I paid close attention to the music that the school band played because I enjoyed it. I enjoyed the music of Karl King, Chicago, Abba, Fleetwood Mac, Earth, Wind & Fire, and the Symphonic pieces from Beethoven, Bach, and Rachmaninov. In home economics, I learned needle point, macramé, knitting, crocheting, painting, designing clothes, drawing. and sketching. Following others was difficult for me. People following me was even more difficult because I was deemed crazy, but not criminally insane crazy. Wanting more from music; I formed a gospel group at church. Three sets of sisters. Sometimes we were serious and sometimes I was just serious. Our hearts and lifestyles showed in our singing. We later combined with some brothers at the church. I wrote some of the music and lyrics that we sang.

I loved the Lord, but not correctly. I became great at faking happy; I was an angry person. Spiritually, I was in and out of church; with no real relationship with the Lord. Yet, He kept me safe! My foolishness proved to be risky, selfish, rude, and sometimes mean. The words "love" and "I'm sorry" did not come easily to my lips. I usually apologized if I hurt people's feelings; then added that I was not sorry for what I said. My insecurities and self-esteem were shaky. I was afraid of fighting, because of my thrill for violence. I was scared of what I may do to the other person. One girl attempted to bully me in school and I always imagined biting off parts of her body and spiting them in her face with confidence. She would touch my food during lunch. One day I just slapped her face just as the bell rang to go to class. I told her that I had to go to class and ran off. Eventually, we became friends.

My virginity was gone in eleventh grade. It was like I misplaced something personal and it was gone forever. It was a horrible event. Love was not involved. It was just something to do that I had not done before. So, it was an experience that I just had to get out of the way. I decided that if that was what sex was about, I would do without it for a

19

while. I sought after drinking, clubbing, and, drugs to escape the responsibilities of adulthood. I was getting bored and people started expecting me to do something strange, comment rudely, or just be brutally honest. I did not like being predictable. I wanted to shock people.   Still, I found that writing was a more satisfying way of expressing my violent thoughts which were all over the place. Jesus still kept my mind.

I decided that my parents were too strict, so instead of college, I joined the Army and was "being all that I could be," during my short stay, those five months and fourteen days, basic training was easy. I was still writing for mental security. What I was going to school for is not what I signed up for. My feet were not army material. I was released on an Honorable Medical Discharge.

Shortly after my discharge, my mother was fussing at all of us on the way to church. I asked if she was finished because it was getting ridiculous. She reached to slap me, and I grabbed her wrist and pushed back. She got quiet and I released her. That was the last time she ever attempted to hit me. It was disrespectful on some type of level. She probably thought about killing me and tossing me out of the car. I apologized to her later that day.

Adulthood

I had my first child at twenty-four. and then another two years later; then another. Their fathers were not a part of their lives. I was unstable mentally carrying the second one. Being pregnant and not married was not a good look in church or for my parents. My family for some reason did not understand why I was a mental wreck but, they were the ones judging and having conversations about me; I expected that from the church. I saw the glances they gave me and their judgmental rulings over me. Folks and family made my decision of giving up my child easy; but, then they could not deal with my decision. At church, I had wondered why my position in the choir was taken away because, they saw that I was pregnant. Clearly if you preach about all sin being the same, then why was lying, gossiping, prevalent fornication, drinking, perversion, and adultery given passes. I guessed then that seeing a sin, and knowing a sin were different. My parents moved and left the house to me and my siblings. We were laughed at and mocked. The expectation was that the children were supposed to leave and not the parents! Rules and regulations for church will never work because of favoritism, fickleness, and the rule-makers are usually the rule-breakers. A relationship with Jesus makes all the difference in the world. I never suffered from church-hurt; maybe people hurt, but not church-hurt. There is no job-hurt, neighborhood-hurt, or club hurt. So, why focus on a building-hurt? Unless a brick hit you or another part of the building: let's be clear: people hurt people! Buildings do not hurt people.

I ended up keeping my second child. After her birth my parents took her until I felt better. My oldest daughter did not understand why her sister did not come home. I explained to her that I could not take care of her. And, with the faith of a child she said, "let's pray and ask Jesus to help us so, she can come home." We got on our knees and prayed for strength and a right mind to take care of both of them. I picked up my second daughter shortly after that. The third pregnancy was a breeze because, I had concluded that only God gives life and only He can take life. My children were gifts and not a curse. I understand that the Lord turned my sin around for good. Giving them away was not the answer to my problems. So, I put my children in the Lord's hands which was a good idea because post-partum depression is real. During bath time I washed them in the sink or in the tub with a level of water so low that it would be impossible to drown them. I always imagined drowning them. I did not want to go into a daze while washing them and drown my children. I called it "Miriam Prevention." I knew what I was capable of, so, I made arrangements and plans to combat my own destructive desires. In my hands they were cared for, but Jesus taught me how to love my children. One afternoon, for curiosity's sake, I decided to smoke crack. This happened when my youngest child was around three or four years old. What a life changing disaster that was! I asked a drug user about the side-affects. She laughed at me. A few hours later she brought some over. I asked about the ingredients. She laughed at me again. She sat down, and we talked about her life. I thought she was thin because of her build. My life turned upside down!

Being a mother was something that I neglected while doing drugs. By the time I started paying attention, during my life on crack, about one year, I was down to 97 pounds. During my stint with this mind-altering drug, I experienced some life changing events. I was in my first fight; I beat up a woman. I was attacked, and threatened at gunpoint, shot at, robbed, threatened again at knife-point. and involved in other illegal acts. My children were placed in my parents' care. I was heartbroken and alone. In my devastation, I prayed and asked the Lord to take the taste for crack away. Immediately, the Lord took that want for crack away. Thank God! I wrote a poem concerning freedom in this storm called "No Longer Walking in Addiction, I'm Abounding in Deliverance."

*I was never arrested or hospitalized.   When you are not thinking of God, He is still thinking of you!

No Longer Walking in Addiction,
I'm Abounding in Deliverance

I struggled with addictions that staggered my life. The afflictions of their predictions were causing restrictions and conflictions during this particular night.

My conscious was no longer responsive to the plan that was meant, but the best defense is the essence that dwells in this flesh. So, in that dark hour, as I prayed alone, soul to Savior; a footstool to His throne, my soul brought forth the identity of that which is keeping me. I'm no longer an addict. I claim victory. I've gotten back to the Adam and Eve of things. You know, before the fruit brought knowledge into the scheme of things. Praising and worshipping Him and never ceasing for a care and receiving all entitlements because you know, I'm His heir.

I'm focused and determined with my peripherals blinded. My faith is a disciplined behavior; it may be bent, but not blind sided. Deliverance got to the root of all things masked. The whys, the how's, the needs; and then I realized it came to pass.

As dawn repeats with not a day counted or measured; Hello! My name is Miriam and I have been delivered. "Being an addict is a constant fight but being delivered is constant liberation."

Miriam Whitehead-Brice

Bill

The social worker on the case explained to me that if I refused rehab then I could not be around my children. I do not frown upon rehabilitation. I just knew it was not for me. I had lost my children, possessions, apartment, friends, and self-esteem, but not Jesus. With the mindset of starting over, I wanted to further my education, so I started going to a Technology school. At that time, I was homeless and staying at friends' houses until my welcome was worn out. Then a seemingly nice man asked me to stay with him while I was getting myself together. We will just call him Bill. My mind was not in a really good place. I never really lived with a man before, I missed many days of school and finally dropped out. He asked me to move with him to Salisbury, Maryland where I was sadly introduced to Domestic Violence.

Having been mentally and physically abused, I sought comfort in drinking, smoking cigarettes, and marijuana. Bill would promise me that he would take me to see my children. I would get dressed and excited, but when we got near, the bridge on the way, he would pull out a fishing pole to fish and I did not get to see my children. He ignored my pleading and crying. Sadly, I can relate to other women in abusive situations now. I did not tell my family and friends because I feared for their safety and was also embarrassed that I was in this situation.

One day after he went to work I left and moved into a shelter. At the shelter, I would call my children. They did not know I was at a shelter. I called Bill and told him where I was when he asked. I fell for his constant lies as he promised to do better. He came to the shelter making a scene. So, I was asked me to leave. I left with him. We visited his parents in North Carolina. I told his mother that he was abusive. Her response was that her husband beat her for 30 years. I had stepped into a generational abuse system. His mother just did not care. I think she told him I was leaving him. Her husband sat in front of

25

the television with a lifeless stare as if he was unaware that I existed. I told her I was leaving him. He would constantly deceive me. I kept hoping that he would change his mind. worse and one That night he snatched me violently from in front of the television. He yelled, I cursed; I slapped, he punched; I threatened his life, he laughed, and we went to bed! After a week or two went by my mother and children came to visit. He pretended to be "Prince Charming." It crushed me to see them leave. I promised them that we would all be back together soon. After they left, Bill promised that he would kill me and bury me in the back yard. I promised him that I would kill him first. He shoved me and left the house for a while. Arguing and fighting became a daily occurrence. I secretly loaded the rifles in the house. I also strategically hid knifes in every room for easy access. I feared the worst but stayed there. I could not go anywhere. Then he allowed me to go to a church of his choice. I asked the church for help. They just prayed for me and drove me back home.

A woman from church would call me, but her husband told her not to get involved with me. I even called the police station and asked them if I could stay the night there. The officer said they were not a hotel. I guess they wanted me to press charges against Bill. I had opportunities to press charges, but I never did. I had become an expert at saying, "everything is fine." My oldest daughter had changed and took on the role of mommy by constantly telling my mother what her sister and brother wanted and how to treat them. It was heart breaking. I had a flashback of my father telling my mother that they were financially able to take care of the children. She called social services anyway to get help and that was when I was told I would not be allowed to be around them because of my refusal to go into drug rehab. I blinked my eyes to hold back the tears and anger. I realized that it was selfishness on my part to think that income was enough to take care of them properly. It hurt that I was in this predicament; I would not sacrifice my wants for my children's needs!

My mother had informed the children's school about my life and circumstances. When visiting the girls in their classes, I had to sign in at the school office. The cold, gossipy, and side-eye glances bothered me.   The absolute silence when I showed my ID was maddening. Seeing my girls was more important to me than their nasty thoughts and stares; it felt as though they were assuming that I was going to kidnap them. I had another flashback of the times, the countless times, that I took my oldest to half-a-day kindergarten in the morning only to have her still there at four o'clock. I had smoked away their Christmas money. The guilt had me in tears when I left their school. Before I left, my oldest asked me if I was I coming back. I said, "yes," but, she sadly walked away as if I was lying to her. "My God! What had I done?" I asked God for deliverance. I was a mother without children.

I talked to the Lord and I knew he was listening. I genuinely prayed for a change of heart and mind; sometimes we ask the Lord for change, a rescue, or an exit, and then when He provides it, we do not recognize it because of self-condemnation or our lack of faith. I saw them regularly but, I did not speak to no one about the abuse. My children missed me. I was grateful for their hugs and kisses which I missed. Because of the craziness of the situation, those kisses were rare; I cherished each one. I got a job and Bill renovated a room for me in the city. I was the only female in the building. Bill and I had an argument one night that started with joking around, and, suddenly he pushed me onto the bed so hard that my knees hit my teeth and caused a gash in my knee. The next day I came home from work and my room was trashed. I called Bill on the phone with a hostile attitude. He said that he shot a hole through my television and took a bat and smashed my stereo.

When I asked him about my clothes, he told me that he threw most of them in a furnace. I went to where he lived to confront him; I then threatened his life with a hammer and knife. He laughed and walked away. I left and felt great about the confrontation.   Life seemed to bare down on me like hard steel. I asked the Lord to get me out of this situation. His reply was that He did, I just needed to, in faith, believe that it was already done, and then walk away.

I took a step of faith. I needed money to get my hair done: I wanted to look nice when I visited my children the next time. I asked Bill and he gave me the money. After I got my hair done, I went home to show off my new hairdo. He was very drunk and passed out. I was furious - I started yelling at him. As soon as he jumped up, he started choking me. Bill's brother watched and told him to calm down; he let me go as I gasped for air. Then I punched his head with my fist. I tried to get away quickly, but with every attempt to leave, he would only allow me to get as far as the front door, then he would pull me back and throw me against the walls. This happened about three to five times. Next, he punched me in my throat, aiming for my face. I grabbed for the phone to call the police, but he threw me in a chair and told me to stay like a dog. I was trying to get my breathing in order. I started cursing the day he was born and his name. Rather than intervening, his brother left with a loud slam of the door. I pleaded with Bill to let me leave. On my fifth or sixth attempt to leave, he let me open the door. I yelled and told him that our relationship was over; this was my good-bye forever! I slammed the door. I spotted a police officer sitting in the lot; I just stared at him. I shook off the moment and got in my car. I just drove past his parked police cruiser thinking about reporting the abuse, the court sessions, and facing him again. The whole incident left a bad taste in my mouth; so, I just pulled up my collar hiding the bruise and left. I had finally walked away physically and emotionally. I gathered up what I could from that room of mine in the city and went to my mother's house. She embraced me with tears and I embraced her with a whimpering cry. There, I was home with a blanket of peace covering me like another layer of skin.

When my children came home from daycare and school, all I could do was to wrap my arms of love around them. They asked me if I was staying forever and I answered them with a tearful but strong, "yes." My eldest daughter asked me several times if I would be there when they came home from school. I could not get angry with her for asking because, she was the one most affected by my drug abuse. As I already said, I would take her to kindergarten school, for her half-day of schooling. I would walk her in the morning and never get her in the afternoon. The school would call me, and I had forgotten to pick her up or was so high that I could not get her. Sometimes she was there for hours until my mother picked her up. I realize now I had to prove to her I would always be there for her. Bill did not take me leaving well. Unbeknown to me, he would stalk and harass my family members constantly asking them where I was. Totally ignoring him, I got another job, because life without my children was devastating and was eating away at my heart. Security was my primary aim for both me and my children; I was finally ready to be a mother. A safe environment was now doable. After dwelling in deplorable living conditions, my mother allowed me to come live with her and my children.

One evening, Bill came to my mother's house and attempted to snatch me out of the house when I opened the door. I twisted my arm to get out of his grip, pushed him back and stepped back into the house. I then slammed the storm dorm and locked it. He tried to open it, banged on it and then turned around kicking things off the porch. After that, I never spoke or heard from him again. I was free. I promised myself to never get in that situation again! It took about two years from the time that I started smoking crack, then lost custody of my children, and got locked into an abusive and toxic situation, until I was free. During that whole time, I was never arrested for anything; to God be the glory! I got a job and my own place. My mother told the social worker assigned to our case that she was returning her grandchildren to me. In assessing the situation, the social worker agreed with my mother. I still had to go to court so that I could obtain custody of my children again.

We moved into a one-bedroom apartment. I worked at a local McDonald's and had the support of my family. The Lord was on our side and He made things work out for me and my children. They were happy, but I was not content concerning their living conditions. I worked as hard as I could. I realize now that the Lord was with us the whole time. I now know that Jesus would not give me such precious gifts without giving me the means to take care of them. The Lord made provision.

After that, we moved again into a duplex. It had enough room for all of us and had a backyard with a fence, but I still wanted more for my children. During my children's elementary school years my own violent tendencies had to be addressed. They had (my children) hurt other children physically and my parents had to pay doctor bills for those injuries. My rage issues had to be addressed and the bad memories that came along with them. Love and consistency made things better as they grew. We all found that there was great truths in the old saying that "laughter is good medicine."

My parents took time to take me and my siblings on vacations and visit family members abroad. We went to parks, Disneyland, zoo's, beaches, etc. It was my desire to take my children places: we rode bikes together, and took nature walks, we crossed creeks, played indoor and outdoor games. This took their minds off their pain. It did not erase the hurts, but, it gave them new, good memories to dwell on. We attended church regularly. My sense of humor has been passed down to my children. I told them that when I pass away, I want to be cremated. I told them to cast my ashes in the waters of Montego Bay in the Caribbean. They told me they would dump me in Baltimore's Inner Harbor because, my ashes would not know the difference. I recalled this scripture "...write the vision and make it plain..." (Habakkuk 2:2). I wrote this on a piece of paper: By the time my oldest child goes to middle school, I will be living back in Baltimore County. My house will have a pink bathroom, a tan bathroom, and a green bathroom; it will also have a big basement and backyard. I met a man in the drive-thru at work one day. I was a little harsh to him at first. He pulled off, but then backed up and gave me his phone number. He was attractive, mannerly, and quiet; he was also focused, communicative, and very funny.

My life experience had taught me to question any man who was being pleasant and mannerly. But, my reflection in that mirror of life also needed to remember that I was "fearfully and wondrously made." Sometimes change can be challenging even if it is for the betterment of life. We hit it off, fell in love, and two-and-a-half years later, in June 1997, we got married. He bought me and the children a home in Baltimore County for a wedding present. It had "a pink bathroom on the first floor, a tan bathroom in the basement, and a green bathroom upstairs; also, a big basement and backyard; five bedrooms and a fireplace were added to my dream!" He loved and took care of us. Wow! "...Goodness and mercy... follows me..." (Psalm 23:6)! We went through marriage counseling okay. Two weeks before our wedding; me and my children moved into the new house my husband bought for us. I made my bridesmaids dresses, my girls dresses and the flower bands on their heads, I even made my own wedding gown, I was sewing at my mother's house and, when I made the train for the gown, my mother commented that she finally believes that I was really getting married. I finished sewing everything on the morning of my wedding; I almost collapsed when I realized I had to make a suit for another person!

My mother finished the last suit and I went to sleep for four hours. Another friend of mine also commented with, "I can't believe that you're getting married before me." The church I attended did not expect much out of me because of my former lifestyle. Little did they know that a "prophetic writer" was being groomed, molded, and tried in the fire to come out as pure gold. Some of the people came to my wedding in disbelief – even some of my own family members. A lot of

31

them came because they loved me and wanted to celebrate the occasion with me.

As an adult, I kept meeting men who wanted to dominate and break me. Maybe I was always perceived as a person who needed rescuing. My husband met me when I needed rescuing. I have been down, but I have never been out. There is a difference. My husband and I are being separated by a five-bedroom house with the children gone. The spare bedrooms have been turned into our needful spaces. I need an office and he needs a man cave. Togetherness is still that one bedroom.

"But I fear, lest somehow, as the serpent
deceived Eve by his craftiness, so your minds may
be corrupted from the simplicity that is in Christ"
(2 Corinthians 11.13).

"In my distress I cried to the Lord, And, He heard me"
(Psalm 120.1).

CHAPTER
TWO

I'm What?

One morning in 2000, I woke up and realized that I had been losing weight. As I got ready for work I prayed and thanked the Lord for another day. My right eye was irritated as well; it was driving me crazy. I looked in the mirror and discovered a sty on the inside my eyelid. I decided to go to the doctor's office during my lunch break to get it looked at and taken care of. I was grateful for my job and flexible hours. I was also thankful that my husband had great medical insurance. In addition to the sty, I had a slight headache, so I ate something before my headache got worse. The food did not help the headache go away.

At Work

At work I greeted everyone. Then I asked my boss if I could go to the doctor's at lunch time. My boss noticed that my eye was swollen and red. I went to the doctor's office at the appointed hour. I told my boss that I would be back in about an hour. My headache was getting worse over my right eye area. I had no idea what was going on. I started worrying and praying; then praying and worrying. Doing both proves you are unstable. Prayer is enough; it works without the worry! What I knew was that my head was pounding; the pain was excruciating!

At the Doctor's Office

I arrived at the doctor's office and there were just two other people waiting. I told the receptionist that I was not okay. My head was pounding. My eye was burning. I was rocking back and forth. "I have a sty in my eyelid that is starting to really bother my eyesight."

Impatiently, I asked how long I was going to have to wait? The receptionist told me that I had about a twenty-minute wait.

Exam Room 3

While I sat there waiting, my scalp started itching. The nurse told me that my body temperature was elevated, and that my blood pressure was a little high. I knew my pressure was always low, and I was always cold. I knew something was wrong! I told the nurse that my pressure was up, because of my headache, but I could not so easily explain away the fever. A few minutes later, the doctor came in to see me. I explained to the doctor what was going on. I had a bump inside of my eyelid and now it felt like two or three. Examining me the doctor asked about the bumps on my scalp and on the right side of my face. I was not aware of that! The doctor told me he would be back in a minute. Worry and questions took control of my emotions and mood. The first doctor came back with another doctor.   Both of them stood quite a distance from me. I told them that "my head and eye felt like they were going to explode?" They told me to look in the mirror. When I looked, I started yelling and crying! The upper right side of my face, some of my scalp, and all around my eye looked horrible! I cried, asking the doctors what was wrong with me. I started putting my hand over my right eye because the light was now bothering me. I kept repeating that "my head and eye are going to explode." Sobbing, I said that it felt like it was getting worse!

The doctors stood away from me and said I had shingles. They asked me if I ever I had the chicken pox? I told them that I had the chicken pox when I was in elementary school. They told me that the virus that causes shingles (varicella virus) is the same virus that causes chicken pox, and that once we have been exposed to the varicella virus, it is in our bodies for the rest of our lives. And, with the virus in our bodies, we could get this painful version of the disease as adults. I asked them if I was contagious? They both said yes, at the same time! I could not return to work for a while. I expressed to them that the pain was unbearable!   They gave me a lot of pain medications and something for that horrible rash.

I started crying again and complaining about the burning pain. They said that I might go blind in my right eye because of nerve damage! They gave me Valtrex for the shingles virus, which is also used for herpes and also caused by the varicella virus.   In my husband's germophobic arrogance, he yelled that he paid too much for health insurance for me to look like that. That just made me cry even more. Later the doctors could not understand why I was not blind in that eye.

Many Months Later

A few months later, I had a sinus infection that lingered too long, and I was still losing weight. My primary care physician referred me to an otolaryngologist (ear, nose, and throat doctor). The specialist looked in my nose and noted that I had a deviated septum. He went on to tell me that my lymph nodes were swollen. Then, to my horror, he sat back and said he often saw the same problems in HIV/AIDS patients. He asked if I had been tested for HIV. At that point, I almost fainted. Tears welled up in my eyes as I told him "no!" My mind started racing in every direction. What if my children had it? Did my husband give it to me? Or, did I give it to him? Who? What? Why?

The drive home seemed to last forever. I went to a clinic the next day, in the city, to get tested. I gave the clinic a fake name. In my mind, if the test came back negative, my name did not need to appear in anyone's database or system. At the time, that made sense to me! I became anxious, weary, and agitated. When did this happen to me? Have I had it for a long time? I saw articles, but I never really read them. I heard things on television but, I never really paid attention. I saw the movie Philadelphia.   Would my body look like that?   Spotted with sores, leaking and bleeding, the loss of weight, and the way the main character was treated; it was horrible. No, no, no! I would shake my head and my body was screaming, "No!" Somehow, I was comforted by the Lord. He gave me peace and I was able to sleep.

But, when I woke the next morning the rants, hollers, doubts, and negative thoughts of confinement started all over again. The word HIV kept spinning around in my head, and it kept circling around in my thoughts. "Jesus where are you!?!?" Back then, it took two weeks for the results of an HIV test to come in. Two weeks came faster than I wanted it to. While waiting in the clinic, I started noticing how people looked. I wondered if they were HIV positive or had full blown AIDS. I paid attention to their skin color, their weight, and their skin blemishes. Just then I realized that I was gnawing on my fingernails.

When they called me by the name I had given them a chill ran down my back. The counselor looked sorrowful as I heard the words, "You are HIV positive." "I'm what?" I mumbled!

I wondered how I had to live? Then the woman said, "Your CD4 count is almost near AIDS. We caught it in time."
"Hmm" I thought!

The counselor asked me if I used intravenous drugs. I said no with a weak and squeaky voice. You were probably infected three to five years ago by the looks of the progression of the disease. Then she questioned me about unprotected sex. I said that I had but, that I could not think of who. All of my partners looked healthy. The counselor kept talking, but my brain had already shut down. My conscious mind was gone but, my body was still present. "I'm what?" kept running through my mind. I called my husband immediately. I cried and cried. My ability to speak was gone.

My breath became pants as my strength left me. My husband immediately came to the clinic. He was very nervous, but he still managed to embrace me tightly. He assured me that everything would be okay. He got tested. I questioned his rationality. Two more weeks had gone by. The whole time, I was on pins and needles; aggravated, angry, anxious, worried, and just an all-around mess! The word HIV made me sick and gave me a headache. And yet, the Lord blanketed my calamity with peace. My husband's test was negative. When we got the news, it seemed as if the whole world went quiet. My husband recalled our wedding vows. "In sickness and in health." He said he loved me and would try his best to keep me alive as long as possible. He held me and squeezed some security back into me. Because my mother had abused me as a child, I was determined to cause problems between her and my father. I wanted him to divorce her. Was I now reaping what I had sown as a child? Maybe I was getting what I deserved. At that moment condemnation replaced chastisement. I felt doom and gloom hovering over me, and not grace and mercy. "Why me?" I could not believe that sentence rang through my head. Was the curtain closing on my life? I felt alone and wanted to hide.

"But, He was wounded for our transgressions,
He was bruised for our iniquities;
The chastisement for our peace was upon Him,
And, by His stripes we are healed" (Isaiah 53.5)

CHAPTER
THREE

Potholes in Life's Roadways

There have been times when mental and physical abuse were a part of my life; these times have occurred during both my childhood and my adulthood. I have tried to self-analyze. I understand and agree with what the scriptures say, "He who spares his rod hates his son, but he who loves him disciplines him promptly" (Proverbs 13:24). But, bruised muscles, damaged mindsets, burnt fingers, and broken hearts are unacceptable. And, never hearing an apology for when a parent has crossed the line between punishment and abuse is not what that scripture meant. As I recall, those times in my life were horrible, but, survival happened. These days, I walk in victory and freedom has been achieved! My mother and I have a great relationship now. I even have respect for my mom. I understand that abuses in her own background were never addressed. As her hurts laid dormant and unhealed, emotional circumstances brought the abuse back out of hibernation. Did extension cords, vacuum pipes, belts, and slaps have to be the consequences for lighting candles, exhibiting a smart-mouth, mistreatment of my siblings, disobedience, and a total disliking of my mother? Whether the answer to that question is yes or no is not what is most important; what is being told here is liberating.

I lit some candles in the window sill. My mother said that I could have started a fire. And yes, stubborn me did it again; so, she wrestled me and placed my fingers in the fire on top of the stove until she thought I might blister or pass out from pain. My siblings and I did not commit crimes – we were just mischievous in the house; sometimes we were noisy when mom wanted to sleep. It is amazing how I cannot remember what I did wrong most of the times but, I remember the punishments. She threw water in my face to wake me up if I was not up when she was up and ready. When it came to arguments, mom had to have the last word. That was a real control issue. When we played games, we had to play so that she would win. That rule was put in place because of some board games and tennis. One board game, in particular, required quick reflexes. She placed a wooden spoon on the table and dared us to scrape her finger while trying to put the game pieces in places. It got quiet, then we all laughed. If you were not fast enough, your fingers might get scraped, and mom's fingers always got scraped. We still recognized that spoon and played with caution.

We would go to the tennis court. One time I was mad at her, so I caught myself teaching her a lesson. Wherever we played tennis, I would hit the ball in the opposite corner from where she was setting up. Mom was running non-stop trying to get the ball until she ran out of breath. She paused and told me that if I did not hit the ball to her that she was not going to play.

Yes, she took us places and played games. This is how I learned to mask my feelings. I pretended to like going places, playing games, and talking about topics that only interested my mother. As a child I had hatred in my heart. I became a talkative person with no filters. I was vengeful and patient with my verbal attacks. We could only talk on the phone for three minutes before she would hang up the phone.

My mom's over-the-top reactions were not limited to just games and conversations. If we did not clean our rooms, she threw our clothes out into the backyard. When it was bedtime, I would have hatred on my heart along with the bad dreams. When the school bus dropped us off, the other children could see our backyard. If clothes were all over the yard they would laugh and say, the "Whitehead's won't be coming outside today." When it was time to beat us, she would close the doors and windows but, the neighbors still heard us screaming and crying. These days, I have a thick skin and do not embarrass easily because of this.

I never called the police on her because my siblings constantly begged me not to call. My wrist is still lumped on the side that my mother hit me with the vacuum pipe. She always wanted the last word, and, if she did not get the last word my face got it. During my first pregnancy my mom told my friends not to celebrate my sin with a baby shower. I did not find that out until many years later. She was religious, self-righteous, wrong, and wayward; and someday I believed she was going to get it right. The neighbors, relatives, and folks down at church knew that we were being beaten horribly. Our sense of humor clouded their judgments and we were just deemed lovable, crazy, and funny. We are great now. After my childhood years, my anger issues became dormant and only extremely emotional stressors brought them out. Violence was intriguing to me. Communication has been the key for change. Today, our relationship is based on forgiveness, understanding, and love. I will protect, fight, and go to bat for my mother.

A Message for Mothers and Daughters

I did not understand, nor did I know love. My mother would say, "I love you," but, the words went unheard because they were matched with beatings. What kind of love was that? Maybe I was selfish. Maybe she had anger issues. Maybe the Lord took me specifically on that journey so that someone who is presently living in hatred, wallowing in pride, fixated on fear, or just plain old disgusted with their mother needed to read this. "I love my mother despite everything. I have moved on. I have forgiven her and have asked the Lord for forgiveness because of my past ungodly thoughts towards my mother. When I prayed and asked the Lord to change her, He told me I had to ask Him to change me! I am to accept her change, apology, past and present circumstances and to allow Him to do the healing; He is much better at that than I am anyway. I got the courage to tell my mother that I felt this way and she was moved, hurt, and apologetic. The communication barriers for me were pride, fear of an unforeseen response, and hurt because I just might not be able to move past my own past. If anyone of you have mother issues, please move past it. Your mother is your mother. Hurt mothers, admit that the shackles are broken, and step up and out for love's sake. If stubbornness is the culprit, remember you are releasing baggage, weight, burdens or heaviness! And, when those things are gone, you will find release from your past. At least the Lord can say that you did your part! Tomorrow is not promised!

What is Love is To Me

Love is a sacrifice of emotions;
You want to give it but, at the same time it is a cherished feeling you
want to guard.
Love is not I, I, I.
It is not even "my way."
It is thoughtful order without a stagnant border!
It is that taste of memorable soup.
Your grandmother seasons it to perfection
But, you like mom's because... it is mom's.
I was spoiled, hard-headed, selfish, solicitous, and silly.
Then I was synthetic, robotic, and callous.
Then I was caring, empathetic, grateful, and a crybaby.
Finally, I find myself determined, edgy, creative, attentive, and
beautiful. Thinking of others is not hard when you do it for good.
Humans are supposed to love with intent emotion.
Some kind of way it spirals into a conventional ride on a boundless
cloud without emotional ties.
Yet, it grieves us with loss.
If you can survive this brain scheming, heart tampering, and
physiological twisting;
you can call love your own. I have chosen to occupy my love in all of
the above, and I think I got it. Right when I gave birth and said,
"I do".

"Casting all you care on Him: for He cares for you" (1 Peter 5.7).

"Be ye angry and sin not: Let not the sun go down upon your wrath" (Ephesians 4.26)

CHAPTER
FOUR

Psychologically Speaking

I went to a reputable hospital for HIV. I heard that their clinic was nice, and that the doctors were pleasant. My husband went with me. Initially, I was distracted by the appearances of the other patients. I asked to be scheduled last when everybody was gone. They respected my request. I was always the last and only patient at the end of the day. The amount of the virus (viral load) in my system was high. My CD4 count, which is a count of the antibodies that fight off the disease, was about four hundred. Two hundred means you have moved from being HIV infected to having AIDS. I was told about the different medications, symptoms, and what to expect concerning my health. This was a nightmare! I was on edge. While the physician was talking, I burst into tears. Reality had struck me like a lightning bolt. There I was being instructed on how to live through this disease that I thought would never land on my doorstep. My husband held my hand and I wriggled it loose. An angry tone spilled out my mouth when I asked, "how long do I have to live?" I wanted to live, but how was I going to?

My faith and fate did not match. My husband bent and placed his elbows on his knees and buried his face in his hands. Then, he sat back up and gasped for air. He asked me to calm down. The doctor suggested that I attend support groups; I agreed with a reluctant disposition. This caused the doctor to question me about telling the truth and keeping in good communication with her. She instructed us to pay attention to our bodies and from now on; condoms must be used at all times during sex. My eyes rolled back in my head and I mumbled about never having sex again. My husband sat there with his hands on his knees shaking his head in disbelief. It was then that I was informed about a program. I am generally a decent dresser and my appearance always had others thinking that everything was alright. No one could visibly see the torment, frustration, hurt, and sad feelings that I was experiencing on the inside. It was as if I was a walking battlefield. I was disgusted for putting myself in this predicament. I did not know why I thought that I was somehow exempt from HIV or AIDS. The doctor commented that I looked nice on the outside. I rolled my eyes! I could not be mad at the world because I knew that this disease was one hundred percent preventable. Now, I felt careless and I was spiraling into depression. I told my family soon after I found out and they were deeply concerned about my well-being. I did not tell my children right away and threatened anyone who would dare to tell them. I was worried about them worrying about me. I wanted them to be happy and go to school with no unnecessary concerns. I told some close friends and they told their close friends and so on... None of them openly rejected me. I was my own worst enemy. Every time that my husband went to get blood work done I cried. Since he was exposed to HIV he had to get tested a couple of times. Every time he went to have blood work drawn, it felt like the first time I told him. Being devastated became a common emotion.

I started going to support groups and seeing an on-site psychologist. The psychologist convinced me to see a psychiatrist. So, I scheduled an appointment to see a psychiatrist. I was told that I had anxiety issues and was bipolar with psychotic tendencies. I now had a psychiatric chart as well as a medical chart! I felt unstable and masked my feelings like an expert! I was put on psychotropic medications. The medicines made me feel drowsy and lethargic all the time. I had no time to think about depression. I would say that sleeping was the closest that I could get to death and I was comfortable sleeping my life away. Also, when you are asleep you are not thinking about problems. I was a walking wreck. Sleep became my escape! My family and husband were not in agreement with my medication regimen; they thought that the medicine was making me more depressed. The HIV medication was causing me to hallucinate during the night. I started sleep walking around the house, holding conversations with myself, and making phone calls at 3 and 4 o'clock in the morning with whoever I could get a hold of at that time of the night. My children became suspicious. They asked me what was wrong? I told them comforting lies. They accepted the lies for the moment. My mother, who has a degree in psychology suggested that I see a different psychiatrist. She was worried that I was over-medicated. I was on Seroquel (an anti-depressant used in treating psychosis and bipolar disorders), Abilify (an anti-depressant, dopamine agonist most often used in treating bipolar disorder and major depression), Doxepin (a tricyclic anti-depressant used primarily to treat major depressive and anxiety disorders), Trazodone (yet another anti-depressant used to treat both major depression and anxiety disorders) and six hundred milligrams of Lithium (used in combination with other anti-depressant drugs and used to reduce the risk of suicidal ideations). As you can see, there were a lot of similar drugs being administered to address the same symptoms.

One psychiatrist asked me why black people were so paranoid? The rude question alone could cause anyone to become paranoid! Needless to say, that was our last meeting. She deemed me a danger to myself and society. I slit my wrist one evening. It was like looking at a bystander cut my lower arm two inches up and down. After realizing what I had done, I drove myself to the hospital. I was hospitalized for three days in a psychiatric facility. I asked the nurse, "why did I have to go to the mental ward because I did not cut my wrist from side to side?" The nurse told me that the way I cut it was the correct way. I just mumbled that I had not read any instruction manual; I just cut it. I then told them that I was over medicated, and that I wanted to live. During my hospitalization, my children came to see me, but my husband could not understand why I had attempted suicide. I believe he was struggling to understand my situation and could not bring himself to visit me in the hospital. It was too much for him. I was furious and called him selfish during a phone conversation. I still said, "I love you" to him. Upon my release, I made an appointment to change my HIV medication. I stopped taking them. This is referred to as a medicine holiday. At the doctor's office I had changed and felt a little more relaxed in that office. I was put on a "medicine holiday." until I was mentally fit to take my medication. Although my CD4 count was higher and my viral load lower, my stability played a major factor in controlling the HIV. Taking medication was never my strong suit. Some medicines I just took when I felt like retreating from the world; that was pretty often.

I decided to get another psychiatrist's opinion of me and he said that I looked "Seroquelized," (if that is even a word, but it was what he said to me). After seeing and speaking with him more diagnoses were added on like Obsessive Compulsive Disorder and more psychotic labels. I felt more comfortable with the new doctor. Consequently, I opened-up more and got to the root of my anger issues and hurt feelings. Coping became a familiar and relaxing word. I was placed on a less severe medicine regimen and my mental health started stabilizing. My HIV medication was changed and "doable." I now faced life, with less sleep! Worrying still lingered, but, was later conquered. Medication compliance was something I had to get used to. It was a discipline thing. I asked my mother about the Lord healing me. She just said, "either pray and take the medication, or pray and don't take the medication." Her advice was not very helpful. So, I prayed, and the Lord answered, basically saying to me that He provides us with resources; He also told me, "take the medicine, but, know that I'm still the one keeping you.

"I can do all things through Christ who strengthens me"
(Philippians 4:13).

CHAPTER
FIVE

Learning Me

The medical clinic that I attended had a pleasant program. I was always asked if I was a counselor because of my appearance. I would tell them that I was a client also. I met a woman, we can call her Celia, who paid close attention to me. Celia told me, to get out of myself and live. Then during lunch, she asked me if I had some money. I said, "yes." She told me that the Red Cross was teaching an HIV/AIDS Teacher and Instructor Course. After taking the course I would be certified to teach and instruct others concerning HIV/AIDS. She also told me that I would learn more about the disease that I have, and how to handle and manage it better. I agreed and took the course. Two other people and I took the class. We let the class know that we were infected with the disease. No one openly treated us differently. As usual, I had no problems blending in with my classmates. I was comfortable and well-liked by the instructors as well. I went from a B student to an A student and earned an A on my final exam.

I enrolled in the Leadership Empowerment and Advocacy Participation program (L.E.A.P.). Publicly speaking about my disease had become second nature to me in the L.E.A.P. program. During that time in the program, I was informed about the other groups that were involved with HIV/AIDS that helped those infected and affected with HIV/AIDS. I joined a number of other support groups and let my voice be known. Since I wrote poetry, I wrote a poem called "Woman of Victory." HIV now meant something different to me and I was feeling one hundred percent better about my life. I had truly cast all my cares to God and moved forward. I wrote another poem called "Why chance it?" I felt that this poem would come across better when it came to a different audience. After praying and having that heal me please conversation with the Lord. God's answer was: "I am all powerful! It's not that I cannot heal you, but you will be one of those examples of how you can be kept and still live with this thorn in your side. This isn't for you; your testimony is for others to endure this walk. I will get the glory out of your life. Wow! His grace is sufficient! Amen and okay!"

In time, my mother and I had become friends; and there was nothing that we would not do for each other. When I think back to my early twenties, my mother told me that it took a long time for her to forgive me for what I had done. That was not a clear statement because I had done so many things; I needed clarity. My thoughts were dizzy trying to circle around the turmoil that she had put me through. I chose to leave it alone. One evening we were all laughing in the living room when my mother said, "if I pulled out a belt right now, Miriam would be the only one to stand here the others would run." There was an awkward silence, then, we all laughed.

If me and my mother have a disagreement these days, we agree to disagree, and we move on in love. Saying I apologize is much easier now because we actually mean it. I call her and help out at her job. Communication with my father was difficult because, he was always traveling. Our communication is always sincere. But, I did have to learn how to communicate with men. Sleeping with men was easy, conversing with them was not. Me being HIV positive has shed some light in the dark places of my life. I have grown so much emotionally and mentally. I face my tomorrows with an understanding that I have no control over tomorrow. Forgiveness and repentance are a daily thing for those circumstances that happen daily. I dwell in Freedom and Liberty. I now understand that when I met my husband I was in an immature place in my life. I was struggling as a single mom with three children.   I was needy and mentally and financially unstable. I guess that I had the appearance of a drowning victim needing to be rescued.   Better financial decisions could have prevented me from creating unnecessary debts. He said at that time that women should not pay bills. He suggested that I get a job to keep "change in my pocket." I was happy about not having to worry about bills anymore. He wanted to be my rescuer always, but that meant that I had to be drowning, always. As I matured and became more stable, positively purposefully, stronger spiritually; we worked it out. He is still HIV negative and we are still together after twenty-one years of marriage!

Woman of Victory

Being Stigmatized and ostracized, through my
eyes see what I've seen.
Being labeled dirty and irresponsible; is it possible to be hopeful in a
world that constantly throws stones?
You pretend to be prayerful with those masks and gloves on!
Are you scared of me? Does my particular
situation cause your mind to roam?
Guess what, in all actuality, reality has hit home.
Infected and affected you can't ignore the pain.
Homosexual or Heterosexual it isn't prejudice and you can't escape the
stain. I was categorized as a statistic and numbered as a loss.
I've been treated less than standard
and ignored like a second thought.
The strength of my self-worth can't be measured or barcoded.
The difference in my life has been turned into a testimony.
Depression is behind me; the closet door is open.
This child of God is no longer a facade; the spirit of fear has been
broken. I'm suited up for a battle
that doesn't involve flesh and blood.
As my soul lies in this bed of clay I'm victorious.
I'm still here for a reason, living in my season,
and passing this message to another;
There is "Life After Diagnosis" and don't accept the scarlet letter.
Lean on His everlasting arms and step out on faith.

Recognize your support system and know that deliverance brings
difference.
I've risen to the occasion of:
His Internal Vision in me. I'm focused on that relationship. As for the
world's notions, well, that's a distraction,
And
I
Don't
Surrender, to it.

Miriam Whitehead-Brice

Why Chance It?

I am no longer living careless treating life as the wind;
Or wandering to and fro giving my life to him, it, and them.
I was struck by the results of mythical thinking:
"I'm Superman, I'm Wonder Woman;
I'm the clock that will keep on ticking."

Now, quarantined by Stigmas, because of living life Las Vegas style;
Taking chances and just giving condoms small glances.
You see, celibacy was not on my mind.
I treated my body like a game of roulette.

It was also like sticking my hand in a bad magician's hat.
I'm carrying a treasure unaware of its measure because I've just got
my mind on some right now pleasure.
Not knowing the outcome, ignorant to the pre-cum,
Wow, if I had just used a condom!

I shared untamed fluids with goals of no boundaries,
Rushing the introduction of, "slow death meet ovaries."
I had the mindset of; it won't happen to me, because of the color of my
skin, my sexual preference, or just this one time, - again.

Now that I've arrived with HIV in my medical folder,
I've got to tell the next person and as I share I become bolder.
I didn't think I was going to make it at first, acceptance was a battle,
but I paused for a moment
And Jesus said, "this, you can handle!"

Little girl, young man, teenager, adult, and seniors change your
methods of thinking and change your modes of tolerance.
I challenge you to open your mind to self -accountability.

Think of yourself and love yourself. Respect starts with self-
commitment. HIV won't defeat me, And I Don't Surrender to Stigmas
and judgments!

Miriam Whitehead-Brice

"He who is without sin among you, let him throw a stone at her first"
(John 8:7).

CHAPTER
SIX

My Inside Is Out

The Health Insurance Portability & Accountability Act of 1996 (most commonly referred to as HIPAA, but also as PL 104-191 or the Kennedy-Kassebaum- Act) – is the primary medical privacy legislation in the United States and it scares people senseless. Medical professionals would talk to me at normal volumes then suddenly whisper, "HIV/AIDS," when that part of the conversation arose. Even though my volume never changed, their volume would lower noticeably; their eyes would go from left to right and their head would move slightly downward. It became humorous to me. At times, I would just mention HIV just to hear a person's volume change. When I finally told my children their response was, "that's all, we thought it was something serious." They make sure that I take my medications. I told her manager and supervisor at a new job. I did not think the other co-workers needed to know. One day at work, the job had a type of fair. I did not have life insurance, so, I filled out an application. I answered the questions truthfully. I handed the application back to the person behind the table and moved on to another table (this one with jewelry on it). The insurance representative jumped up from behind the table yelling out my name. Her voice was high, excited, and loud. She informed me that I made a mistake on the application. She was noticeably out of breath. She told me that I checked that I was HIV positive; and obviously I was not! The room suddenly got quiet and all of the (nosey) ears in the room were listening; all of the busy-bodies were watching! I said back to her in a semi-loud voice that I apologized, and the representative scratched it off. Immediately, I went to a phone and called the insurance company and told them what had happened and said that their representative needed more sensitivity training.   After taking a payroll deduction out of my pay for the next months, I was surprised when I received a notice of not being qualified for that life insurance.

I had to have blood work done every three months. This was for an update to see if the medicines were working and to make sure other things in my body were okay. It was a little chilly that day, so I had on long sleeves. After my name was called, I went back to get my blood drawn. I saw the phlebotomist pick up her orders; this woman started huffing and puffing, sighing loudly, and slamming vials and paperwork around! I knew at that moment that the phlebotomist undoubtedly assumed that I had contracted HIV from shared needles. I guess that she that thought that finding a vein would be difficult. Quietly, I rolled up my sleeves to reveal gorgeous, thick, and visible veins; I could hear an audible sigh of relief from the phlebotomist. I am known to have a quick wit. Total strangers – people who do not really know me, feel that they had a right to ask me invasive questions. My intentional and biting responses showed no signs of being filtered. This time wisdom took a hold of me and I just blurted out that I became HIV positive from unprotected sex. It was hard for me to say anything else. The woman thanked me without an apology. She told me that she needed to hear that. I turned my head and held back the tears.

It took about five years to get to that point in my life where tears would not fall for pity's sake. As people found out, the word rejection became like a callous on a construction workers hand. I got used to it, sometimes I   deliberately yelled, "Yes, I'm HIV positive. Can we move on now?" At other times, I ignored people's nasty looks and stares. I went to a certain clinic for pain. When the receptionist read my paper work she would display a negative attitude.   I watched as the receptionist read my diagnosis to the other women in the front area. All the other patients that came into the office after me had been seen and left. I noticed that a different group was now with me waiting to be seen. I also realized that an hour-and-a-half had gone by. I questioned the receptionist and the other women giggled. Anger boiled up in me as I blatantly stood up beside the receptionist desk and stared at her until the woman became uncomfortable. The doctor came out and I got very loud and my words were not pleasant. The doctor made an excuse for their actions at the front desk. That was the last time I attended that clinic. I have nothing good to say about that particular office.

I was told that I was an advocate and activist. If I thought that someone in my vicinity was being treated differently, because they had HIV/AIDS my brain (and mouth) would automatically go into lawyer mode. I am aware of my rights and their rights; I am also aware of the correct protocols and procedures. If this is the definition of advocate and activist, then I wear that title with pride.

Since my diagnosis, my relationship with the Lord has become much more personal. I had finished a book of spiritual poetry called, Gifted Words: Poems of Promise and Praise. I was going to have my first book signing. At first, I was going to reveal to my audience that I was HIV positive. At that point, many people still did not know. I told my best friend and youngest daughter that I had changed my mind because fear and doubt had reared its ugly head. To them that reason was just not good enough and that "the show must go on."

After speaking with my husband, my confidence boosted to another level. My husband's approval meant the world to me! That first book signing went very well. I read my poetry and let everyone there know about my health. Since being diagnosed with HIV, which, by that time, was undetectable with a very low viral load, my doctors have found many other health problems with me. Sometimes, the doctors wondered and commented on how I managed to look so well. What a Stigmas flag that is! At that book signing I let them know about my HIV. I told the audience that since 2000 the doctors have also diagnosed me with lupus, fibromyalgia, and phlebitis, I need a completely new right knee, I have had trigeminal neuralgia, asthma, and six screws and rods put in my lower spine from degenerative disc disease. In addition, I am bipolar with anxiety issues and have had a history of attempted suicide, obsessive compulsive disorder, human papilloma virus, a torn rotator cuff, and cataracts in both eyes. Shall I go on? There are also endometriosis, bursitis, problems with my coccyx bone, three cysts on my left kneecap and osteoporosis, peripheral autonomic neuralgia, sinus problems and acid reflux.

People at the book signing gasped and made "wow!" sounds. I finished up with asking them, "but, aren't I beautiful?" There was an electric applause and a standing ovation among the crowd. Since then, I have a new knee, both of my shoulders have been repaired again; I have four new screws and two latches placed in my upper neck (spine), and four toes that have been repaired. God gets the glory out of my life!

"For I consider that the sufferings of this present time are not worthy to be compared with the glory which shall be revealed in us" (Romans 8:18).

My smile and sense of humor stands strong.

CHAPTER
SEVEN

Life After Diagnosis

I was the client at a medical facility and was hired there as an HIV/AIDS consultant. During my work and attendance there, I was on the board and the president of the Clients' Advocacy Board (C.A.B.). I also joined two phenomenal organizations. The first organization consisted of women 50 years and older. This organization is called Older Woman Embracing Life (OWEL); it is phenomenal. We meet once a month and learn something new to strengthen, incite, promote, and persevere whether infected or affected with HIV/AIDS. I wrote their creed. It was during one of their meetings that they I became aware that they needed some people to volunteer for a project for the state of Maryland. I was interviewed and became one of the four people to be a spokesmodel for HIV/AIDS campaign called "HIV Stops with Me." My full photo and HIV diagnosis date was placed on buses and billboards throughout the state of Maryland. I was interviewed on television's Grace and Glory, and the web from London, England for "truthloader.com" twice. I have been reading my poetry up and down the east coast of the United States. I am looking forward to venturing on the west coast.

Contact me! When I spoke at an awareness festival in Washington, DC, I was deemed to be an HIV/AIDS activist. I have been inducted into 20/20 Leading Woman Society in Atlanta, Georgia. When March's Funeral Homes (in Baltimore) Celebration of Community Workers Calendar came out in 2014, my mom, my sister and I were featured for the month of May. The women in my family are part of the "Whitehead Women's Wellness Institute." We want to see people live up to their maximum capacities.   I am a minister of the Gospel of Jesus Christ and have been to colleges, churches, and numerous venues speaking about "Life After Diagnosis" which is one of my registered trade names. I am a published author. To date, I have completed six books. One book is called My Grandma Is HIV Positive and I am working on six more plus one anthology of my works. I wrote the musical play "Skits of Praise." I wrote the music and lyrics. The play debuted in January 2016. I am a chaplain with the Baltimore City Police Department Chaplaincy Program.   Additionally, I am in the grassroots stage of establishing a new non-profit organization called Share Your Story to Empower Many (SYSTEM). SYSTEM is one of my many trade names.   My byline says, "We seek to create a pulse in statistically flat-lined mindsets and communities."

I have been invited to participate in a panel for the Delta's at the Washington (DC) Press Club about HIV/AIDS, given lectures at the Delta Sorority on World AIDS Day and at the Zeta Phi Building in Maryland concerning HIV/AIDS and Seniors, and have guest lectured at Coppin State University. I spoke at Beautiful Gate in Delaware for National Women and Girls HIV/AIDS Awareness Day, was interviewed by TruthLoader.com from London, England about "Serodiscordant Couples," and did a project with a reporter from Canada.   I was interviewed on WEAA radio at Morgan State University and Radio One. I spoke at the "Legends and Youngun's" Conference for OWEL and am a member of the HIV Planning Group for the state of Maryland. In addition to all of that, I have spoken and recited poetry at various churches, conferences, health fairs, and schools – spreading the message of Life After Diagnosis. I am currently working on a book that I'm making into a play I wrote call "Rhythms of Unheard Voices" which will debut in March of 2019. I will bring awareness to women and men unfairly imprisoned and judged for killing or have attempted to kill their abusive partners or spouses.

I have seen that people can also be diagnosed as a nuisance or outcast too. I tell them that they are just "set apart for a higher calling." There are some people who are just going to attempt to knock you down; they are only comfortable in negative mode. Someone once asked me how long it had been since I used drugs. I answered by telling them that my former failures do not count. When this happens, I ask them when the last time was that they lied or gossiped? That usually puts a stop to their negativity. I wonder why it is that only some sins have to be measured with a start and stop dates? As far as I am concerned, I am delivered and, that counts for a whole lot more than the fact that I was once bound. I believe that you can still live and be a productive member within your family and community no matter what the diagnosis. I never want people to give up; I am proof that life's problems can be overcome if you set your mind to it. When I see a caterpillar (which is what some folks call it), I call it a beautiful moth or butterfly. I see past its worm stage. I attempt to see beyond what my limited eyes show me.
I think everyone has potential and I quote,

"Sometimes another's belief in someone could create a systematic release in that one."

- Miriam Whitehead-Brice

There are many people walking around unaware that they are HIV positive. Some just do not care. Stigmas are used to create barriers and closeted conversations. Singing about sex seems to be popular, especially in heavily populated groups of people that are infected by HIV/AIDS. Pay attention to what you listen to because music has an effect on you. In my opinion the phrase "know your status" promotes Stigmas also. That phrase is not used for any other disease!

Walking into a room full of people who know I am is HIV positive used to bother me. Now, I realize that it was not only me being uncomfortable. Lots of people see me and are reminded of their indiscretions or sexual encounters where they did not use protection (I have asked them). I do not want anyone to feel uncomfortable, so, I tell them to know the facts about HIV/AIDS and get tested.

My viral load is low (undetectable) and my CD4 count is not near 200 (which doctors say is the threshold between being HIV positive and having AIDS. My children and grandchildren are all HIV negative.

Seniors are the new group of people getting infected. No one is comfortable in asking seniors, "Are you using condoms?" This is especially true when that senior happens to be a parent or grandparents. Seniors can live well and long with HIV/AIDS by getting tested. Age is not a reason to ignore any diseases, especially if you are still sexually active. By the way, as was my case, shingles may be a good reason to get tested!   Every day you should be an inspiration to someone or be inspired by someone. That will keep you attentive of your surroundings.

You should look out for my upcoming television program Life After Diagnoses on LIFE VISION (a Roku box is needed). In the program, I point out that Jesus is real, and I have found favor in the Lord! Are you living your best life after any diagnosis?

Love Lifted Me

I was rolling around in the muck and mire of life.
I dwelt in the hatred that pressed upon my heart.
My emotions were on play time as a theatrical cloud fell over me
And, I played a significant part.
I fell into a compromising state even though I knew it wasn't right.
There was no sense of hope.
There was no peace in sight.
Disappointment had saturated my expectations.
The maturity of my mental stability became stagnant in direction.
There was no scent of joy.
The bounds of condemnation were tight.
The cuffs of aggravation strangled my outward appearance.
I was familiar with left and displayed an allergic reaction to right.
An anchor of depression kept me still in one place.
Shackles of despair were holding on to me like a tourniquet.
I was on the edge of sorrow.
I was at the end of my rope.
I heard a voice calling me.
There was a stirring deep down in my soul.
Right there in the thickness of my anguish; right there on the path towards death.
The Lord provided an answer.
He said, "you're going through, so keep your eyes on the exit."
Then suddenly the spiraling chains of fear were lifted.
Suddenly the shackles broke free.
Immediately I walked into freedom.
Love lifted me.
Then my heart got lighter.
Then was I provided liberty's keys.
It was then that I realized that love was always there.
The problem was me.
You see, I was caught up in a whirlwind of emotional stress.
Illnesses had me downtrodden, but, Jesus deemed me not forgotten.
Jesus embraces, society rejects.
Love lifted the burdens.

Love paralyzed this flesh.
Love greeted happiness.
Love took the sting out of death.
Love showed me the miracle of what freedom should be.
Love came down to where I was. "Love lifted me."

Have Faith and Change!

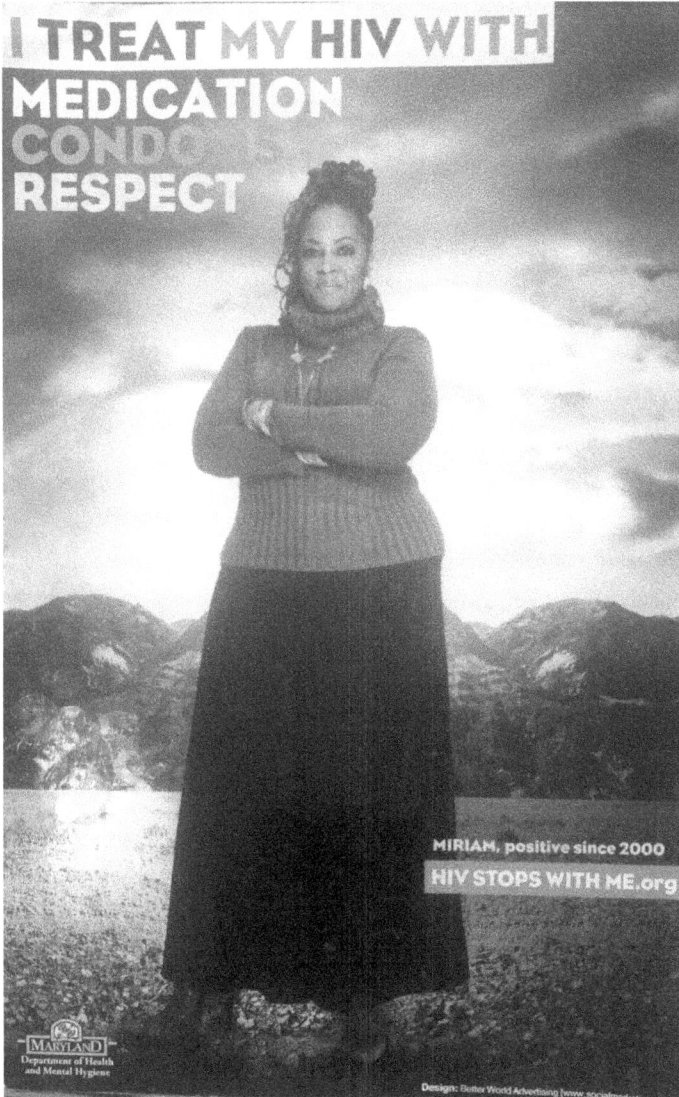

I am one of the four Spokes Models.
This is my spokes model picture from the
"HIV STOPS WITH ME CAMPAIGN"

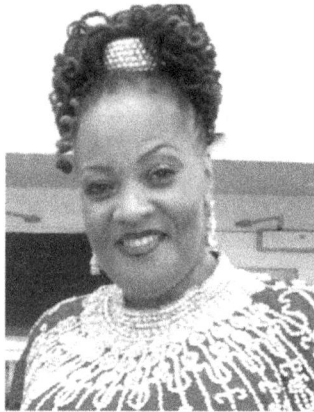

I was inducted into the 2020 Leading Women Society
in Atlanta, Georgia.

www.ingramcontent.com/pod-product-compliance
Lightning Source LLC
Chambersburg PA
CBHW031140270326
41931CD00007B/633